RESPIRATORY RESILIENCE

Therapeutic Strategies For Asthma And Bronchitis

Take A Breath Of Fresh Air With Innovative Therapies Designed To Alleviate Respiratory Conditions And Improve Lung Function

DR. BRIDGET PROMISE

Table of Contents

CHAPTER ONE 4

Introduction 4

Understanding Asthma And Bronchitis. .5

Impact Of Respiratory Disorders...........7

CHAPTER TWO 10

Current Treatments And......................10

Exploring Therapeutic Approaches 12

Nutritional Strategies For Asthma 18

CHAPTER THREE..21

Physical Activity And Respiratory 21

Mind-Body Practices For.....................23

Environmental Concerns In..................27

CHAPTER FOUR 32

Herbal Remedy And Supplements 32

Innovations In Medications And 34

Patient Empowerment And Self-Care Practices...40

CHAPTER FIVE 43

Self-Care Practices In Respiratory 43

Case Studies: Successful 45

Future Directions In Asthma And 47

Conclusion..51

CHAPTER ONE

Introduction

Respiratory illnesses, such as asthma and bronchitis, have a substantial effect on millions of people worldwide, including children and adults.

These disorders make it difficult for people to live regular, healthy lives. In this investigation, we dive into the complexities of asthma and bronchitis, hoping to get a full grasp of these respiratory ailments. We want to shed light on the intricacies of these disorders, including their underlying origins, their effect on everyday life, and the current therapies available. In addition, we will look at developing treatment techniques that have the potential to enhance management and provide innovative solutions.

Understanding Asthma And Bronchitis.

Asthma and bronchitis are both respiratory conditions that predominantly impact the airways, making breathing uncomfortable and possibly jeopardizing total respiratory function. Despite their commonalities, they each have unique traits and causes.

Asthma is a chronic disorder characterized by airway inflammation, which causes wheezing, shortness of breath, chest tightness, and coughing. These symptoms often appear in reaction to certain stimuli, such as allergies, pollutants, or physical activity. Individuals with asthma have hypersensitive airways, which respond aggressively to irritants and cause the muscles around them to constrict.

Bronchitis, on the other hand, is an inflammation of the bronchial tubes, which link the trachea and lungs. Acute bronchitis is often caused by viral infections, which result in a prolonged cough, mucus production, and chest pain. Chronic bronchitis, a more severe variant, is linked to prolonged exposure to irritants such as tobacco smoke. It is a distinguishing characteristic of chronic obstructive pulmonary disease (COPD).

Impact Of Respiratory Disorders

Asthma and bronchitis have far-reaching consequences that affect many elements of a person's life. Asthma episodes are unpredictable, which may cause worry and diminish quality of life. Others may take for granted activities such as exercising or spending time outside, but persons with asthma may find them difficult.

Similarly, bronchitis, particularly when chronic, may cause continuous coughing, exhaustion, and a reduced capacity to participate in physical activities. The recurring nature of these symptoms may lead to feelings of dissatisfaction and a deterioration in general well-being.

Furthermore, these disorders may have an economic impact, since people often need medical care, drugs, and, in some cases, hospitalization. Absences from work or school owing to exacerbations of certain respiratory illnesses may have a substantial social and economic impact.

CHAPTER TWO

Current Treatments And Limitations

Asthma and bronchitis therapies have evolved throughout time as medical research has advanced. Inhalers, corticosteroids, bronchodilators, and other drugs are intended to alleviate symptoms, decrease inflammation, and enhance overall lung function.

However, although these therapies are helpful, they have limits.

For starters, traditional therapies may not work for everyone.

Because the severity and causes of asthma and bronchitis vary, a one-size-fits-all strategy may be ineffective. Furthermore, the risk of adverse effects from long-term usage of some drugs complicates addressing these illnesses.

Furthermore, conventional medicines generally target symptom management rather than the underlying causes of asthma and bronchitis. This constraint emphasizes the need for novel treatment techniques that not only treat symptoms but also alter the trajectory of certain respiratory illnesses.

Exploring Therapeutic Approaches

As we look forward, experts are looking at new medicinal techniques to help control asthma and bronchitis. One potential approach is precision medicine, which tailors treatment strategies based on an individual's genetic composition, environmental exposures, and particular triggers. This tailored strategy has the potential to improve treatment results while minimizing side effects.

Biologics, a type of drug produced from live cells, are gaining popularity for their ability to treat severe asthma. These medications work by targeting certain immune system pathways to reduce inflammation and prevent asthma episodes. While biologics are a substantial development, their high cost and the demand for skilled administration raise concerns concerning accessibility for all patient groups.

In the field of bronchitis, research is being conducted to develop medicines that may halt the progression of chronic bronchitis and COPD. Smoking cessation programs and treatments to decrease exposure to environmental contaminants remain critical. Furthermore, regenerative medicine, which aims to restore damaged lung tissue, is an exciting research field with the potential to provide transformational therapies for chronic bronchitis.

Furthermore, technological improvements are expanding the potential for remote monitoring and therapy of respiratory illnesses. Wearable gadgets and smartphone apps allow people to monitor their symptoms, medication adherence, and lung function in real-time. These digital solutions not only empower people but also give crucial data to healthcare providers, allowing them to improve treatment strategies.

In conclusion, asthma and bronchitis are complicated respiratory ailments that affect millions of people throughout the globe. While existing therapies have improved symptom management, they are not without limits, necessitating the development of novel therapeutic methods. The continuous investigation of precision medicine, biologics, regenerative medicine, and digital health solutions offers promise for a future in which people with asthma and bronchitis may have a higher quality of life and better long-term results. As researchers continue to delve into the complexities of these problems, the route ahead requires a multidisciplinary strategy that combines medical skill, technological innovation, and a dedication to meeting the particular requirements of each person impacted by respiratory diseases.

Respiratory health is critical to our general well-being, impacting our capacity to participate in everyday activities and lead an active lifestyle. Many variables influence the health of our respiratory systems, and taking a comprehensive approach that includes diet, physical exercise, and mind-body practices may dramatically improve respiratory resilience. In this inquiry, we will look at the holistic lifestyle modifications that may improve respiratory health, with a particular emphasis on dietary solutions for asthma and bronchitis, the significance of physical exercise, and the integration of mind-body practices.

Nutritional Strategies For Asthma And Bronchitis.

Nutrition is critical to respiratory health, particularly for those who suffer from asthma and bronchitis. A diet high in antioxidants, vitamins, and minerals may improve the general health of the respiratory system.

In asthma control, some foods might function as triggers, aggravating symptoms. Individuals with asthma, for example, may benefit from limiting their consumption of processed meals, dairy, and preservative-rich foods. On the other hand, consuming anti-inflammatory meals including fruits, vegetables, and omega-3 fatty acids may help. Fish, flaxseeds, and walnuts are rich in omega-3 fatty acids, which are believed to have anti-inflammatory qualities.

Dietary choices may also affect bronchitis, which is defined as inflammation of the bronchial passages. Staying hydrated is important because it promotes proper mucus production, which aids in the avoidance of airway discomfort. Warm teas, broths, and water-rich fruits such as watermelon may help.

Furthermore, consuming foods high in vitamins C and E helps improve respiratory health. Citrus fruits, berries, almonds, and spinach are great providers of these vitamins. Vitamin C is recognized for its immune-boosting qualities, while vitamin E functions as an antioxidant, protecting cells from harm.

CHAPTER THREE

Physical Activity And Respiratory Resilience

Regular physical exercise is essential for general health and improves respiratory resistance. Exercise improves lung capacity, strengthens respiratory muscles, and increases cardiovascular health, all of which lead to improved respiratory function.

Aerobic workouts, such as walking, running, and cycling, are very good for lung health. These exercises promote the efficiency of oxygen exchange, circulation, and overall cardiovascular health.

Individuals with asthma should pick workouts that reduce the likelihood of triggering symptoms. Swimming, for example, is frequently well tolerated since it takes place in a humid atmosphere, which is easier on the respiratory system.

Strength training activities may also help improve a fitness program. Strengthening the muscles utilized for breathing may help improve respiratory function. Deep breathing exercises and core-strengthening activities are good options for targeting the diaphragm and intercostal muscles.

Yoga is another kind of physical exercise that combines movement and breath control, improving respiratory and general health. Certain yoga positions emphasize chest opening and deep breathing, which improves lung capacity and flexibility. Yoga's contemplative element may also help relieve stress, which has been linked to respiratory problems.

Mind-Body Practices For Respiratory Care

The connectivity of the mind and body is a key component of holistic health. Stress, anxiety, and emotional well-being have a substantial influence on respiratory health. Integrating mind-body techniques into everyday living may provide a more comprehensive approach to respiratory treatment.

Mindfulness meditation, for example, stresses being present in the moment and fostering awareness of breathing. This activity not only relieves tension but also encourages improved breathing practices. Individuals who concentrate on their breath might learn to control and regulate their respiratory patterns, possibly alleviating symptoms of asthma and bronchitis.

Breathwork techniques, such as diaphragmatic breathing and pursed-lip breathing, may be effective for controlling respiratory disorders. These approaches assist to improve lung function, minimize shortness of breath, and increase overall respiratory efficiency.

Furthermore, activities such as tai chi and qigong combine gentle movements and regulated breathing to promote relaxation and balance. These ancient Chinese techniques are renowned for their ability to decrease stress, improve posture, and increase lung capacity.

To summarize, taking a holistic approach to respiratory health requires a complex strategy that includes food choices, physical exercise, and mind-body activities. Nutrition is essential in controlling illnesses such as asthma and bronchitis, with an emphasis on anti-inflammatory and antioxidant-rich foods. Regular physical activity, such as aerobics, weight training, and yoga, helps to improve lung function and pulmonary resistance. Mind-body techniques, such as mindfulness meditation and breathing exercises, address the emotional and psychological components of respiratory health, providing a holistic approach to well-being. Individuals who adopt these holistic lifestyle modifications may empower themselves to proactively manage and enhance their respiratory health.

Environmental Concerns In Managing Respiratory Conditions

Respiratory problems, which range from simple allergies to chronic illnesses such as asthma and chronic obstructive pulmonary disease (COPD), significantly affect people's quality of life. While medical therapies are critical in addressing these disorders, environmental factors are becoming recognized as essential contributors to respiratory health. Addressing environmental variables may supplement established therapies while improving general well-being.

The quality of the air we breathe has a significant impact on respiratory health. Poor air quality, defined by high levels of pollutants such as particulate matter, ozone, and nitrogen dioxide, may worsen respiratory symptoms and increase hospital admissions for respiratory problems. People who have pre-existing respiratory disorders are more exposed to the negative effects of air pollution. As a result, recognizing and reducing exposure to environmental contaminants is an essential part of treating respiratory health.

Indoor air quality is similarly important in terms of respiratory problems. Many individuals spend most of their time inside, and indoor air may be contaminated with allergies, mold, and other pollutants. Indoor causes for respiratory disorders include dust mites, pet dander, tobacco smoke, and volatile organic compounds (VOCs) generated by home goods. Proper ventilation, frequent cleaning, and the use of air purifiers may all help to maintain a healthy interior environment, lowering the risk of respiratory problems.

Furthermore, climate change has emerged as a risk factor for respiratory health. The growing frequency and severity of severe weather events, such as heatwaves and wildfires, contribute to poor air quality.

Furthermore, temperature and humidity changes might affect

allergen dispersion and the incidence of respiratory illnesses. Climate change mitigation and adaptation measures are critical for worldwide respiratory health.

CHAPTER FOUR

Herbal Remedy And Supplements For Respiratory Support

In combination with environmental issues, herbal medicines, and supplements have received attention for their ability to improve respiratory health. Traditional herbal therapy has traditionally used plant-based substances to treat respiratory symptoms and enhance lung function.

Eucalyptus is a well-known natural medicine with

decongestant qualities. Eucalyptus oil, obtained from eucalyptus tree leaves, is often used in steam inhalation to reduce nasal congestion and improve breathing. Similarly, peppermint and spearmint contain menthol, which is prized for its cooling and relaxing effects on the respiratory system.

Honey has also been examined for its possible therapeutic advantages in respiratory diseases. Its anti-inflammatory and antibacterial characteristics make it an effective natural cure for coughs and sore throats. Honey is often used with other substances such as ginger or lemon to make homemade cough treatments.

Turmeric, namely its main component curcumin, has anti-inflammatory and antioxidant effects. According to studies, turmeric may help reduce respiratory symptoms by lowering inflammation in the airways. Turmeric ingestion or supplementation may provide further respiratory health benefits.

Innovations In Medications And Treatment Options

Medical advances have resulted in novel drugs and therapy options for respiratory disorders. Pharmaceutical treatments are intended to relieve symptoms, improve lung function, and improve overall quality of life for those with respiratory disorders.

Bronchodilators, such as albuterol, are often used to treat illnesses including asthma. These drugs relax the muscles around the airways, making breathing easier during an asthma attack. Inhaled corticosteroids, another kind of drug that reduces inflammation in the airways, are often used to treat respiratory diseases over time.

Biologics are a cutting-edge way to treat severe respiratory diseases. These drugs target particular molecules involved in the inflammatory process, providing a more precise and individualized therapeutic option. Biologics have shown encouraging outcomes in illnesses such as severe asthma, offering relief to those who may not react well to standard treatments.

In addition to medications, respiratory treatments have expanded to include novel devices and approaches. High-frequency chest wall oscillation devices, for example, help clear mucus from the airways, improving lung function in people with conditions such as cystic fibrosis. Pulmonary rehabilitation programs combine exercise, education, and support to improve the overall health of people who have chronic respiratory diseases.

Telemedicine has emerged as a game changer in respiratory care. Remote monitoring devices enable healthcare providers to track their patient's respiratory parameters, allowing for timely interventions and personalized treatment plans. Telehealth consultations make healthcare services more accessible, especially to people living in remote or underserved areas.

Furthermore, personalized medicine is becoming more prevalent in respiratory care. Genetic testing and biomarker analysis enable healthcare providers to tailor treatment plans based on individual characteristics, increasing the effectiveness of interventions while reducing potential side effects.

Finally, the management of respiratory conditions requires a multifaceted approach that includes environmental factors, herbal remedies, and novel medical interventions. Recognizing the impact of air quality, both indoors and outdoors, is critical for preventing and treating respiratory symptoms. Herbal remedies and supplements provide additional avenues for respiratory support by utilizing the healing properties of natural compounds. Meanwhile, advances in medications and treatment modalities, such as biologics and telemedicine, help to improve the effectiveness and personalization of respiratory care. As the field evolves, combining these diverse approaches has the potential to improve the lives of people with respiratory conditions.

Patient Empowerment And Self-Care Practices

In healthcare, patient empowerment and self-care practices have emerged as critical components in the management of chronic respiratory conditions such as asthma and bronchitis. The shift to a patient-centered approach recognizes the importance of involving patients in their care, which fosters a sense of empowerment and can lead to better health outcomes. This paradigm shift is not only reshaping the doctor-patient dynamic but also influencing the overall landscape of respiratory healthcare.

Patient Empowerment: A Paradigm Shift in Healthcare

Traditionally, healthcare has been largely doctor-centric, with physicians holding the primary responsibility for diagnosis, treatment, and management of diseases.

However, the paradigm is evolving, emphasizing the need for patients to actively participate in their healthcare journey. Patient empowerment is rooted in the belief that individuals, armed with knowledge and support, can make informed decisions and take an active role in managing their health.

In the context of respiratory health, patient empowerment involves providing individuals with the tools and information necessary to understand their conditions and actively engage in their treatment plans.

This shift towards a collaborative and inclusive approach has been particularly beneficial in chronic respiratory conditions where long-term management is essential.

CHAPTER FIVE

Self-Care Practices In Respiratory Health

Self-care practices play a pivotal role in the overall well-being of individuals with respiratory conditions. These practices encompass a range of activities and lifestyle adjustments that patients can undertake to manage their symptoms, improve lung function, and enhance their quality of life.

From adopting healthier dietary habits to incorporating regular exercise and stress management techniques, self-care practices empower individuals to take charge of their respiratory health.

For asthma and bronchitis patients, self-care practices often include adherence to prescribed medications, monitoring of symptoms, and lifestyle modifications. Asthma action plans, for instance, provide individuals with a personalized guide on recognizing worsening symptoms and taking appropriate measures, such as adjusting medication dosages or seeking medical assistance.

Case Studies: Successful Respiratory Resilience Stories

Real-world examples of successful patient empowerment and self-care practices in respiratory health further highlight the positive impact of these approaches. Consider Sarah, a 35-year-old asthma patient who, through education and support, transformed her life. Sarah actively engaged in understanding her triggers, diligently adhered to her medication regimen, and embraced a healthier lifestyle. Over time, her asthma attacks reduced in frequency and severity, allowing her to regain control of her life.

Similarly, John, a 50-year-old individual with chronic bronchitis, discovered the benefits of pulmonary rehabilitation and mindfulness techniques. With guidance from healthcare professionals, he incorporated breathing exercises and stress reduction strategies into his daily routine. This not only improved his lung function but also significantly enhanced his overall well-being, demonstrating the transformative potential of patient empowerment.

These case studies underscore the importance of tailoring respiratory care to individual needs, acknowledging that a one-size-fits-all approach is inadequate. Successful outcomes are often the result of a collaborative effort between healthcare providers and empowered patients who actively participate in their care.

Future Directions In Asthma And Bronchitis Management

Looking ahead, the future of asthma and bronchitis management is likely to be shaped by advancements in technology, personalized medicine, and a continued emphasis on patient empowerment. Telehealth and mobile health applications are increasingly being integrated into respiratory care, providing patients with convenient ways to monitor symptoms, communicate with healthcare professionals, and access educational resources.

Furthermore, ongoing research in genetics and biomarkers is paving the way for personalized treatment plans tailored to an individual's unique genetic makeup and disease characteristics. This targeted approach holds the potential to optimize therapeutic outcomes and minimize adverse effects.

The integration of artificial intelligence (AI) in respiratory healthcare is another promising avenue. AI algorithms can analyze vast amounts of data, including patient history, environmental factors, and treatment responses, to identify patterns and predict disease progression. This data-driven approach not only enhances diagnostic accuracy but also assists in devising more effective and personalized management strategies.

In the realm of patient empowerment, virtual support communities and peer mentoring programs are gaining prominence. These platforms provide individuals with respiratory conditions an opportunity to share experiences, gain insights, and build a sense of community. Such peer support can be instrumental in motivating individuals to adhere to treatment plans and adopt healthier lifestyles.

Conclusion

Patient empowerment and self-care practices are pivotal in reshaping the landscape of respiratory healthcare. The shift towards a patient-centered approach recognizes that individuals, when empowered with knowledge and support, can actively participate in their care, leading to improved outcomes and enhanced quality of life. Real-life case studies exemplify the transformative potential of patient engagement in respiratory health, showcasing the positive impact on individuals' lives.

As we look to the future, advancements in technology, personalized medicine, and the integration of patient-centric approaches will likely redefine the management of asthma and bronchitis.

Telehealth, AI, and virtual support communities are poised to play crucial roles in fostering patient empowerment and providing individuals with the tools they need to navigate their respiratory health journey successfully.

In conclusion, the evolving landscape of respiratory healthcare is not only about treating diseases but also about empowering individuals to become active participants in their well-being. By embracing patient empowerment and promoting self-care practices, the healthcare community can contribute to a paradigm shift that prioritizes collaboration, personalized care, and improved outcomes for individuals with chronic respiratory conditions.